DIABETIC RENAL SMOOTHIE COOKBOOK FOR BEGINNERS

Flavorful Blends for Blood Sugar Balance and Kidney Health With Low Potassium, Sodium, and Phosphorus Recipes

By

Dr. Donna Matias

Table of Contents

Introduction to Diabetic Renal Smoothies

Welcome to the world of Diabetic Renal Smoothies, a comprehensive guide designed to support individuals managing both diabetes and renal health concerns through delicious and nutritious smoothie recipes.

Living with diabetes and kidney disease can present unique dietary challenges, but with the right guidance and recipes, it's possible to enjoy flavorful and satisfying smoothies while promoting optimal health.

Understanding Diabetes and Kidney Health

Diabetes and kidney health are intricately connected, with diabetes being one of the leading causes of kidney disease. To understand how these conditions intersect, it's essential to grasp the fundamentals of both diabetes and kidney health.

Diabetes:

Diabetes is a chronic condition characterized by elevated blood sugar levels due to the body's inability to produce or effectively use insulin, the hormone responsible for regulating blood sugar. There are primary types of diabetes:

• **Type 1 Diabetes:** Occurs when the immune system mistakenly attacks and destroys insulin-producing cells in the pancreas, leading to insulin deficiency.

• **Type 2 Diabetes:** Develops when the body becomes resistant to insulin or fails to produce enough insulin to meet its needs.

In either type of diabetes, persistently high blood sugar levels can damage various organs and tissues over time, including the kidneys.

Kidney Health:

The kidneys play a crucial role in filtering waste products, excess fluids, and toxins from the bloodstream, regulating electrolyte balance, and producing hormones that control blood pressure and red blood cell production. Chronic kidney disease (CKD) occurs when the kidneys become damaged and can no longer function properly. CKD progresses through stages, ranging from mild kidney damage to end-stage renal disease (ESRD), requiring dialysis or kidney transplantation for survival.

The Connection Between Diabetes and Kidney Health:

Diabetes is the leading cause of kidney disease, accounting for approximately 44% of new cases of kidney failure in the United States. High blood sugar levels associated with diabetes can damage the small blood vessels and filters in the kidneys, impairing their ability to remove waste and toxins from the body efficiently. Over time, this damage can lead to CKD and, ultimately, kidney failure if left untreated.

Managing Diabetes and Kidney Health:

Managing diabetes and kidney health requires a comprehensive approach that includes:

• **Blood Sugar Control:** Maintaining target blood sugar levels through medication, diet, exercise, and regular monitoring is crucial for preventing kidney damage and slowing the progression of CKD.

- **Blood Pressure Management:** Controlling high blood pressure through lifestyle modifications and medication can help protect the kidneys from further damage.

- **Healthy Lifestyle Habits:** Adopting a healthy lifestyle that includes a balanced diet, regular exercise, maintaining a healthy weight, avoiding tobacco use, and limiting alcohol consumption can support overall kidney health and diabetes management.

- **Regular Monitoring:** Individuals with diabetes should undergo regular screening tests, including blood tests to assess kidney function (e.g., serum creatinine, estimated glomerular filtration rate) and urine tests to check for proteinuria (protein in the urine), a sign of kidney damage.

Importance of Nutrition in Managing Diabetes and Renal Health

Nutrition plays a pivotal role in managing both diabetes and renal health. For individuals navigating the complexities of diabetes alongside kidney disease, making mindful dietary choices is paramount to controlling blood sugar levels, preserving kidney function, and thwarting complications. Here's a detailed exploration of why nutrition holds such significance in managing these conditions:

Blood Sugar Control:

- **Carbohydrate Moderation:** Carbohydrates directly influence blood sugar levels. Opting for complex carbohydrates with a low glycemic index helps mitigate spikes in blood sugar, promoting steadier glucose levels over time.

- **Balanced Meals**: Ensuring meals comprise a mix of carbohydrates, proteins, and healthy fats aids in stabilizing blood sugar, averting drastic fluctuations throughout the day.

- **Portion Management**: Monitoring portion sizes is crucial. It helps in regulating blood sugar levels and forestalling excessive carbohydrate intake, which could otherwise precipitate blood sugar spikes.

Preservation of Kidney Health:

- **Sodium Regulation:** Sodium restriction is pivotal for individuals with kidney disease. Excessive sodium can escalate blood pressure and exacerbate kidney damage. A low-sodium diet aids in curbing fluid retention and reducing blood pressure, thereby alleviating strain on the kidneys.

- **Management of Phosphorus and Potassium:** Monitoring phosphorus and potassium intake is essential. These minerals can accumulate in the bloodstream when kidney function is impaired. Adhering to guidelines for phosphorus and potassium intake helps in mitigating their buildup and preserving kidney function.

Protein Moderation:

- **Protein Quality and Quantity:** Selecting high-quality protein sources and moderating protein intake is vital. It aids in minimizing the burden on the kidneys, as excessive protein consumption can heighten kidney workload and worsen renal function.

Nutrient Density and Balance:

- **Micronutrient-Rich Foods:** Prioritizing foods abundant in essential vitamins and minerals fosters overall health. Opting for nutrient-dense options supports immune function and aids in combatting potential nutrient deficiencies, common in individuals with diabetes and kidney disease.

- **Hydration:** Maintaining adequate hydration is crucial. It supports kidney function, aids in waste elimination, and helps in regulating blood pressure.

Tailored Nutrition and Consultation:

- **Individualized Approach:** Recognizing that dietary needs vary among individuals underscores the importance of personalized nutrition plans. Customizing dietary strategies in collaboration with healthcare providers ensures optimal management of diabetes and renal health.

- **Professional Guidance:** Seeking guidance from registered dietitians or nutritionists with expertise in diabetes and kidney disease facilitates informed decision-making. They provide tailored recommendations and support individuals in navigating dietary challenges effectively.

In essence, prioritizing nutrition in managing diabetes and renal health empowers individuals to proactively safeguard their well-being. By adopting mindful eating habits, making informed dietary choices, and seeking professional guidance, individuals can optimize their nutritional intake and enhance their overall health outcomes.

Overview of Smoothies as a Nutrient-Dense Option

Smoothies have emerged as a popular and convenient choice for individuals seeking a nutrient-dense and wholesome dietary option. These blended beverages offer a myriad of benefits, making them an excellent choice for individuals managing diabetes and renal health concerns. Here's an overview of why smoothies are considered a nutrient-dense option:

1. Nutrient Variety:

Smoothies allow for the incorporation of a diverse array of nutrient-rich ingredients into a single serving. Fruits, vegetables, nuts, seeds, and dairy or plant-based milk alternatives can all be seamlessly blended together, providing a wide spectrum of essential vitamins, minerals, antioxidants, and phytonutrients in one delicious package.

2. Convenient and Portable:

Smoothies offer unparalleled convenience, making them ideal for individuals with busy lifestyles or those on the go. With minimal preparation time required, smoothies can be whipped up quickly and consumed at home, at work, or on the move, ensuring that nutritious options are readily available whenever hunger strikes.

3. Hydration Support:

Many smoothie ingredients, such as fruits and vegetables, have high water content, contributing to hydration levels. Adequate hydration is essential for kidney health and overall well-being, making smoothies an excellent choice for maintaining hydration while enjoying a delicious and satisfying beverage.

4. Fiber-Rich:

Smoothies can be an excellent source of dietary fiber, particularly when incorporating whole fruits, vegetables, and seeds. Fiber plays a crucial role in regulating blood sugar levels, promoting digestive health, and supporting satiety, making smoothies a filling and satisfying option for individuals managing diabetes and renal health concerns.

5. Customizable and Flexible:

One of the most appealing aspects of smoothies is their versatility. Recipes can be easily customized to suit individual preferences, dietary restrictions, and nutritional needs. Whether adjusting the sweetness level, swapping out ingredients, or adding protein or healthy fats, smoothies can be tailored to meet specific dietary requirements with ease.

6. Blood Sugar Control:

When carefully crafted with balanced ingredients, smoothies can support stable blood sugar levels. Choosing low-glycemic index fruits, incorporating protein and healthy fats, and avoiding added sugars can help prevent blood sugar spikes, making smoothies a diabetes-friendly option.

7. Kidney-Friendly Options:

For individuals managing renal health concerns, smoothies can be modified to accommodate dietary restrictions related to sodium, potassium, and phosphorus. Selecting low-potassium fruits and vegetables, using unsweetened milk alternatives, and limiting high-phosphorus additives can help create kidney-friendly smoothies.

Nutritional Guidelines for Diabetic Renal Smoothies

Dietary Restrictions and Considerations

Managing diabetes and renal health requires careful attention to dietary restrictions and considerations to support overall well-being and prevent complications. Here's an overview of key dietary restrictions and considerations for individuals navigating these conditions:

1. Carbohydrate Control:

- **Diabetes:** Monitoring carbohydrate intake is crucial for managing blood sugar levels. Individuals with diabetes often need to limit their carbohydrate intake to prevent spikes in blood sugar.

• **Renal Health:** While carbohydrates themselves are not restricted for kidney health, individuals with kidney disease may need to monitor their carbohydrate intake to manage blood sugar levels and prevent complications associated with diabetes.

2. Sodium Restriction:

• **Diabetes and Renal Health:** Excessive sodium intake can lead to high blood pressure and fluid retention, placing strain on the kidneys and worsening kidney function. Limiting sodium intake is essential for managing blood pressure and preserving kidney health.

3. Potassium and Phosphorus Management:

• **Renal Health:** Individuals with kidney disease may need to restrict their intake of high-potassium and high-phosphorus foods to prevent electrolyte imbalances and complications associated with kidney dysfunction.

• **Diabetes:** While potassium and phosphorus are not typically restricted for individuals with diabetes, those with kidney disease may need to monitor their intake of these minerals to support renal health.

4. Protein Moderation:

• **Renal Health:** Limiting protein intake may be necessary for individuals with advanced kidney disease to reduce the workload on the kidneys and manage waste products effectively.

• **Diabetes:** While protein intake is generally not restricted for individuals with diabetes, choosing high-quality protein sources and moderating intake may be beneficial for overall health and blood sugar management.

5. Fluid Restriction:

• **Renal Health:** In some cases of advanced kidney disease, fluid intake may need to be restricted to prevent fluid overload and complications such as edema and hypertension.

• **Diabetes:** While fluid intake is not typically restricted for individuals with diabetes, staying adequately hydrated is essential for overall health and blood sugar management.

6. Glycemic Index Consideration:

• **Diabetes:** Choosing foods with a lower glycemic index can help prevent rapid spikes in blood sugar levels. Opting for whole grains, fruits, and vegetables with a lower glycemic index can support stable blood sugar control.

7. Individualized Nutrition Plans:

It's essential for individuals with diabetes and kidney disease to work closely with healthcare providers, including registered dietitians or nutritionists, to develop personalized nutrition plans tailored to their specific needs, preferences, and medical history.

By adhering to these dietary restrictions and considerations, individuals can effectively manage their diabetes and renal health, supporting overall well-being and preventing complications associated with these conditions. Collaboration with healthcare professionals ensures that dietary recommendations are personalized and aligned with individual health goals and needs.

Balancing Carbohydrates, Proteins, and Fats

Achieving a balanced diet that includes appropriate amounts of carbohydrates, proteins, and fats is essential for individuals managing diabetes and renal health. By carefully balancing these macronutrients, individuals can support stable blood sugar levels, preserve kidney function, and promote overall well-being. Here's a closer look at the role of carbohydrates, proteins, and fats, along with strategies for achieving balance:

1. Carbohydrates:

Role: Carbohydrates are the body's primary source of energy and have a significant impact on blood sugar levels. Choosing the right types and amounts of carbohydrates is crucial for managing blood sugar levels effectively.

• Strategies:

Focus on complex carbohydrates such as whole grains, fruits, vegetables, and legumes, which provide fiber and essential nutrients while causing less drastic spikes in blood sugar.

Monitor portion sizes and limit intake of refined carbohydrates, sugary snacks, and processed foods, which can lead to rapid increases in blood sugar levels.

2. Proteins:

Role: Proteins are essential for muscle repair and growth, immune function, and hormone production. Incorporating adequate protein into the diet helps maintain muscle mass, support overall health, and promote satiety.

● **Strategies:**

Choose lean protein sources such as poultry, fish, tofu, legumes, and low-fat dairy products to minimize saturated fat intake.

Monitor portion sizes and aim for a moderate intake of protein throughout the day, spreading protein intake evenly across meals and snacks.

3. Fats:

Role: Fats play a crucial role in providing energy, supporting cell growth, and aiding in the absorption of fat-soluble vitamins. Including healthy fats in the diet helps promote heart health and overall well-being.

- **Strategies:**

Prioritize unsaturated fats, including monounsaturated and polyunsaturated fats found in sources such as nuts, seeds, avocados, olive oil, and fatty fish.

Limit saturated fats and trans fats found in processed and fried foods, which can contribute to heart disease and inflammation.

Be mindful of portion sizes and aim for a balanced intake of fats to support overall health without overconsuming calories.

Achieving Balance:

• **Portion Control:** Monitoring portion sizes of carbohydrates, proteins, and fats is crucial for achieving balance and preventing overconsumption of any one macronutrient.

• **Meal Planning:** Planning meals that include a mix of carbohydrates, proteins, and healthy fats helps ensure balanced nutrition and supports stable blood sugar levels.

• **Dietary Variety:** Incorporating a variety of foods from different food groups provides a diverse array of nutrients and helps prevent nutrient deficiencies.

- **Monitoring Blood Sugar:** Regularly monitoring blood sugar levels and adjusting dietary intake as needed in consultation with healthcare providers helps maintain optimal blood sugar control.

By balancing carbohydrates, proteins, and fats in their diet, individuals can support overall health, manage diabetes and renal health effectively, and promote long-term well-being. Consulting with healthcare professionals and registered dietitians can provide personalized guidance and support in achieving dietary balance.

Breakfast Blends:

Berry Breakfast Boost:

Ingredients:

• 1 cup mixed berries. (strawberries, blueberries, raspberries)

• 1 ripe banana

• 1/2 cup plain Greek yogurt

• 1/2 cup almond milk. (or any milk of your choice)

• 1 tablespoon honey or maple syrup (optional)

• Ice cubes (optional)

Preparation:

● Place the mixed berries, banana, Greek yogurt, almond milk, and honey or maple syrup (if using) in a blender.

● Blend on high speed till smooth and creamy.

● If desired, add ice cubes and blend again until well incorporated.

● Pour the smoothie into glasses and serve immediately. Enjoy your Berry Breakfast Boost!

Spinach Banana Power Smoothie:

Ingredients:

- 1 ripe banana

- 1 cup fresh spinach leaves

- 1/2 cup plain Greek yogurt

- 1/2 cup almond milk. (or any milk of your choice)

- 1 tablespoon almond butter

- 1 teaspoon honey or maple syrup. (optional)

- Ice cubes (optional)

Preparation:

- Peel the banana and place it in a blender.

- Add the fresh spinach leaves, Greek yogurt, almond milk, almond butter, and honey or maple syrup (if using) to the blender.

- Blend on high speed until the ingredients are well combined and the smoothie is creamy.

- If desired, add ice cubes and then blend again until smooth.

- Pour the Spinach Banana Power Smoothie into glasses and serve immediately. Enjoy your nutritious and delicious smoothie!

Almond Butter Green Smoothie:

Ingredients:

- 1 cup fresh spinach leaves

- 1/2 ripe avocado

- 1 ripe banana

- 1 tablespoon almond butter

- 1/2 cup almond milk. (or any milk of your choice)

- 1 teaspoon honey or maple syrup. (optional)

- Ice cubes (optional)

Preparation:

● Place the fresh spinach leaves, ripe avocado, banana, almond butter, almond milk, and honey or maple syrup (if using) in a blender.

● Blend on high speed until the ingredients are thoroughly mixed and the smoothie is creamy.

● Add ice cubes if desired and blend again until smooth and well combined.

● Pour the Almond Butter Green Smoothie into glasses and serve immediately. Enjoy the nourishing goodness of this green smoothie!

Peachy Oatmeal Smoothie:

Ingredients:

- 1 ripe peach, pitted and sliced

- 1/2 cup rolled oats

- 1/2 cup plain Greek yogurt

- 1/2 cup almond milk. (or any milk of your choice)

- 1 tablespoon honey or maple syrup

- 1/2 teaspoon vanilla extract

- Ice cubes (optional)

Preparation:

- Place the sliced peach, rolled oats, Greek yogurt, almond milk, honey or maple syrup, and vanilla extract in a blender.

- Blend on high speed until the ingredients are well combined and the smoothie is creamy.

- If the smoothie is too thick, add more almond milk to reach your desired consistency.

- Add ice cubes if desired and blend again until smooth.

- Pour the Peachy Oatmeal Smoothie into glasses and serve immediately. Enjoy this delightful and satisfying smoothie as a nutritious breakfast or snack!

Cinnamon Apple Pie Smoothie:

Ingredients:

- 1 medium apple, cored and diced

- 1/2 ripe banana

- 1/4 cup rolled oats

- 1/2 cup plain Greek yogurt

- 1/2 cup almond milk. (or any milk of your choice)

- 1/2 teaspoon ground cinnamon

- 1 tablespoon honey or maple syrup

- Ice cubes (optional)

Preparation:

• Place the diced apple, banana, rolled oats, Greek yogurt, almond milk, ground cinnamon, and honey or maple syrup in a blender.

• Blend on high speed until the ingredients are thoroughly mixed and the smoothie is creamy.

• If the smoothie is too thick, then add more almond milk to achieve your desired consistency.

• Add ice cubes if desired and blend again until smooth and well combined.

• Pour the Cinnamon Apple Pie Smoothie into glasses and serve immediately. Enjoy the warm flavors of cinnamon and apple in this delicious smoothie!

Carrot Cake Smoothie:

Ingredients:

- 1 large carrot, peeled and chopped

- 1/2 ripe banana

- 1/4 cup rolled oats

- 1/2 cup plain Greek yogurt

- 1/2 cup almond milk. (or any milk of your choice)

- 1 tablespoon almond butter

- 1 tablespoon honey or maple syrup

- 1/2 teaspoon ground cinnamon

- 1/4 teaspoon ground nutmeg

- Ice cubes (optional)

Preparation:

● Place the chopped carrot, banana, rolled oats, Greek yogurt, almond milk, almond butter, honey or maple syrup, ground cinnamon, and ground nutmeg in a blender.

● Blend on high speed until the ingredients are well combined and the smoothie is creamy.

● If the smoothie is too thick, add more almond milk to reach the desired consistency.

● Add ice cubes if desired and blend again until smooth and creamy.

● Pour the Carrot Cake Smoothie into glasses and serve immediately. Enjoy the flavors of carrot cake in this nutritious and satisfying smoothie!

Blueberry Chia Protein Smoothie:

Ingredients:

- 1/2 cup fresh or frozen blueberries

- 1 tablespoon chia seeds

- 1/2 cup plain Greek yogurt

- 1/2 cup almond milk. (or any milk of your choice)

- 1 scoop vanilla protein powder

- 1 tablespoon honey or maple syrup (optional)

- Ice cubes (optional)

Preparation:

- Place the blueberries, chia seeds, Greek yogurt, almond milk, vanilla protein powder, and honey or maple syrup (if using) in a blender.

- Blend on high speed until the ingredients are well combined and the smoothie is creamy.

- If the smoothie is too thick, then add more almond milk to achieve your desired consistency.

- Add ice cubes if desired and blend again until smooth and well combined.

● Pour the Blueberry Chia Protein Smoothie into glasses and serve immediately. Enjoy this protein-packed smoothie as a nutritious breakfast or post-workout refuel!

Kiwi Kale Morning Mix:

Ingredients:

● 1 ripe kiwi, peeled and chopped

● 1 cup chopped kale leaves

● 1/2 ripe banana

● 1/2 cup plain Greek yogurt

● 1/2 cup almond milk. (or any milk of your choice)

● 1 tablespoon honey or maple syrup

- Ice cubes (optional)

Preparation:

- Place the chopped kiwi, kale leaves, banana, Greek yogurt, almond milk, and honey or maple syrup in a blender.

- Blend on high speed until the ingredients are thoroughly mixed and the smoothie is creamy.

- If the smoothie is too thick, then add more almond milk to reach your desired consistency.

- Add ice cubes if desired and blend again until smooth and well combined.

- Pour the Kiwi Kale Morning Mix into glasses and serve immediately. Enjoy this vibrant and refreshing smoothie as a nutrient-packed start to your day!

Citrus Sunshine Smoothie:

Ingredients:

- 1 orange, peeled and segmented

- 1/2 ripe banana

- 1/2 cup pineapple chunks

- 1/2 cup plain Greek yogurt

- 1/2 cup almond milk. (or any milk of your choice)

- 1 tablespoon honey or maple syrup

- Ice cubes (optional)

Preparation:

• Place the orange segments, banana, pineapple chunks, Greek yogurt, almond milk, and honey or maple syrup in a blender.

• Blend on high speed until the ingredients are well combined and the smoothie is creamy.

• If the smoothie is too thick, then add more almond milk to achieve your desired consistency.

• Add ice cubes if desired and blend again until smooth and frothy.

• Pour the Citrus Sunshine Smoothie into glasses and serve immediately. Enjoy the bright and refreshing flavors of citrus in this delightful smoothie!

Mango Coconut Yogurt Smoothie:

Ingredients:

- 1 cup diced mango (fresh or frozen)

- 1/2 cup plain Greek yogurt

- 1/2 cup coconut milk

- 1 tablespoon honey or maple syrup

- 1/2 teaspoon vanilla extract

- Ice cubes (optional)

Preparation:

- Place the diced mango, Greek yogurt, coconut milk, honey or maple syrup, and vanilla extract in a blender.

- Blend on high speed until the ingredients are well combined and the smoothie is creamy.

- If the smoothie is too thick, add more coconut milk to reach the desired consistency.

- Add ice cubes if desired and blend again until smooth and creamy.

- Pour the Mango Coconut Yogurt Smoothie into glasses and serve immediately. Enjoy the tropical flavors of mango and coconut in this delicious and nutritious smoothie!

Energizing Morning Picks:

Green Tea Berry Blast:

Ingredients:

- 1 green tea bag

- 1/2 cup hot water

- 1/2 cup frozen mixed berries. (strawberries, blueberries, raspberries)

- 1/2 ripe banana

- 1/2 cup spinach leaves

- 1/2 cup plain Greek yogurt

- 1 tablespoon honey or maple syrup (optional)

- Ice cubes (optional)

Preparation:

● Steep the green tea bag in hot water for 3-5 minutes to brew a strong tea. Allow it to cool.

● In a blender, combine the brewed green tea (cooled), frozen mixed berries, ripe banana, spinach leaves, Greek yogurt, and honey or maple syrup (if using).

● Blend on high speed till smooth and creamy.

● If the smoothie is too thick, add more water or ice cubes and blend again until desired consistency is reached.

● Pour the Green Tea Berry Blast into glasses and serve immediately. Enjoy the antioxidant-rich goodness of this refreshing smoothie!

Pineapple Turmeric Zest:

Ingredients:

- 1 cup fresh pineapple chunks

- 1/2 teaspoon ground turmeric

- 1/2 teaspoon ground ginger

- 1/2 cup coconut water

- Juice of 1/2 lemon

- 1 tablespoon honey or maple syrup

- Ice cubes (optional)

Preparation:

• Place the fresh pineapple chunks, ground turmeric, ground ginger, coconut water, lemon juice, and honey or maple syrup in a blender.

• Blend on high speed till smooth and well combined.

• If the smoothie is too thick, add more coconut water or ice cubes and blend again until desired consistency is reached.

• Pour the Pineapple Turmeric Zest into glasses and serve immediately. Enjoy the tropical flavors with a zesty twist of turmeric!

Beetroot Berry Energizer:

Ingredients:

• 1 small cooked beetroot, peeled and diced

• 1/2 cup frozen mixed berries. (strawberries, blueberries, raspberries)

• 1/2 cup plain Greek yogurt

1/2 cup almond milk. (or any milk of your choice)

• 1 tablespoon honey or maple syrup

• Ice cubes (optional)

Preparation:

• Place the cooked beetroot, frozen mixed berries, Greek yogurt, almond milk, and honey or maple syrup in a blender.

• Blend on high speed till smooth and creamy.

• If the smoothie is too thick, add more almond milk or ice cubes and blend again until desired consistency is reached.

• Pour the Beetroot Berry Energizer into glasses and serve immediately. Enjoy the vibrant color and energy-boosting benefits of this nutritious smoothie!

Matcha Avocado Delight:

Ingredients:

• 1 teaspoon matcha powder

• 1/2 ripe avocado

- 1/2 cup spinach leaves

- 1/2 cup pineapple chunks

- 1/2 cup coconut water

- 1 tablespoon honey or maple syrup

- Ice cubes (optional)

Preparation:

- In a blender, combine the matcha powder, ripe avocado, spinach leaves, pineapple chunks, coconut water, and honey or maple syrup.

- Blend on high speed till smooth and creamy.

- If the smoothie is too thick, add more coconut water or ice cubes and blend again until desired consistency is reached.

- Pour the Matcha Avocado Delight into glasses and serve immediately. Enjoy the antioxidant-rich goodness and creamy texture of this unique smoothie!

Ginger Pear Refresher:

Ingredients:

- 1 ripe pear, cored and diced

- 1/2-inch piece of fresh ginger, peel it and grate it

- 1/2 cup plain Greek yogurt

- 1/2 cup almond milk. (or any milk of your choice)

- 1 tablespoon honey or maple syrup

- Juice of 1/2 lemon

- Ice cubes (optional)

Preparation:

- Place the diced pear, grated ginger, Greek yogurt, almond milk, honey or maple syrup, and lemon juice in a blender.

- Blend on high speed till smooth and creamy.

- If the smoothie is too thick, then add more almond milk or ice cubes and blend again until desired consistency is reached.

• Pour the Ginger Pear Refresher into glasses and serve immediately. Enjoy the refreshing combination of ginger and pear in this revitalizing smoothie!

Orange Carrot Vitality:

Ingredients:

• 1 large carrot, peeled and chopped

• 1 orange, peeled and segmented

• 1/2 cup plain Greek yogurt

• 1/2 cup almond milk. (or any milk of your choice)

• 1 tablespoon honey or maple syrup

• Ice cubes (optional)

Preparation:

• Place the chopped carrot, orange segments, Greek yogurt, almond milk, and honey or maple syrup in a blender.

• Blend on high speed till smooth and creamy.

• If the smoothie is too thick, add more almond milk or ice cubes and blend again until desired consistency is reached.

• Pour the Orange Carrot Vitality into glasses and serve immediately. Enjoy the vibrant color and citrusy flavor of this invigorating smoothie!

Papaya Mango Sunrise:

Ingredients:

- 1 cup diced papaya

- 1/2 cup diced mango

- 1/2 cup coconut water

- Juice of 1/2 lime

- 1 tablespoon honey or maple syrup

- Ice cubes (optional)

Preparation:

- Place the diced papaya, diced mango, coconut water, lime juice, and honey or maple syrup in a blender.

• Blend on high speed till smooth and well combined.

• If the smoothie is too thick, add more coconut water or ice cubes and blend again until desired consistency is reached.

• Pour the Papaya Mango Sunrise into glasses and serve immediately. Enjoy the tropical flavors and refreshing taste of this sunrise-inspired smoothie!

Spinach Strawberry Kickstart:

Ingredients:

- 1/2 cup fresh spinach leaves

- 1 cup fresh or frozen strawberries

- 1/2 ripe banana

- 1/2 cup plain Greek yogurt

- 1/2 cup almond milk. (or any milk of your choice)

- 1 tablespoon honey or maple syrup

- Ice cubes (optional)

Preparation:

● Place the fresh spinach leaves, strawberries, banana, Greek yogurt, almond milk, and honey or maple syrup in a blender.

● Blend on high speed till smooth and creamy.

● If the smoothie is too thick, add more almond milk or ice cubes and blend again until desired consistency is reached.

● Pour the Spinach Strawberry Kickstart into glasses and serve immediately. Enjoy the refreshing taste and nutrient-packed goodness of this green smoothie!

Banana Walnut Protein Punch:

Ingredients:

- 1 ripe banana

- 1/4 cup walnuts

- 1/2 cup plain Greek yogurt

- 1/2 cup almond milk. (or any milk of your choice)

- 1 scoop vanilla protein powder

- 1 tablespoon honey or maple syrup

- Ice cubes (optional)

Preparation:

• In a blender, combine the ripe banana, walnuts, Greek yogurt, almond milk, vanilla protein powder, and honey or maple syrup.

• Blend on high speed till smooth and creamy.

• If the smoothie is too thick, add more almond milk or ice cubes and blend again until desired consistency is reached.

• Pour the Banana Walnut Protein Punch into glasses and serve immediately. Enjoy the protein-packed goodness and nutty flavor of this satisfying smoothie!

Cranberry Almond Power-Up:

Ingredients:

- 1/2 cup cranberries (fresh or frozen)

- 1/4 cup almonds

- 1/2 cup plain Greek yogurt

- 1/2 cup almond milk. (or any milk of your choice)

- 1 tablespoon honey or maple syrup

- Ice cubes (optional)

Preparation:

• Place the cranberries, almonds, Greek yogurt, almond milk, and honey or maple syrup in a blender.

• Blend on high speed till smooth and creamy.

• If the smoothie is too thick, add more almond milk or ice cubes and blend again until desired consistency is reached.

• Pour the Cranberry Almond Power-Up into glasses and serve immediately. Enjoy the tartness of cranberries and the crunch of almonds in this energizing smoothie!

Refreshing Midday Sips:

Cucumber Mint Cooler:

Ingredients:

- 1 cucumber, peeled and chopped

- Handful of fresh mint leaves

- Juice of 1 lime

- 1 tablespoon honey or maple syrup

- 1 cup cold water

- Ice cubes

- Mint sprigs for garnish (optional)

Preparation:

- In a blender, combine the chopped cucumber, fresh mint leaves, lime juice, honey or maple syrup, and cold water.

- Blend until smooth.

- Strain the mixture through a fine mesh sieve to remove any pulp (optional).

- Pour the cucumber-mint mixture into glasses filled with ice cubes.

- Garnish with mint sprigs if desired.

- Serve immediately and enjoy the refreshing Cucumber Mint Cooler!

Watermelon Basil Splash:

Ingredients:

- 2 cups cubed watermelon

- Handful of fresh basil leaves

- Juice of 1 lime

- 1 tablespoon honey or maple syrup

- 1 cup cold water

- Ice cubes

- Basil leaves and watermelon wedges for garnish (optional)

Preparation:

- In a blender, combine the cubed watermelon, fresh basil leaves, lime juice, honey or maple syrup, and cold water.

- Blend until smooth.

- Strain the mixture through a fine mesh sieve to remove any pulp (optional).

- Pour the watermelon-basil mixture into glasses filled with ice cubes.

- Garnish with basil leaves and watermelon wedges if desired.

- Serve immediately and enjoy the revitalizing Watermelon Basil Splash!

Lemon Ginger Cooler:

Ingredients:

- 1 lemon, juiced

- 1-inch piece of fresh ginger, peeled and grated

- 1 tablespoon honey or maple syrup

- 1 cup cold water

- Ice cubes

• Lemon slices and ginger slices for garnish (optional)

Preparation:

• In a blender, combine the lemon juice, grated ginger, honey or maple syrup, and cold water.

• Blend until well combined.

• Strain the mixture through a fine mesh sieve to remove any pulp (optional).

• Pour the lemon-ginger mixture into glasses filled with ice cubes.

• Garnish with lemon slices and ginger slices if desired.

• Serve immediately and enjoy the invigorating Lemon Ginger Cooler!

Raspberry Lime Sparkler:

Ingredients:

• 1 cup fresh raspberries

• Juice of 2 limes

• 1 tablespoon honey or maple syrup

• 1 cup cold water

• Sparkling water

• Ice cubes

• Fresh raspberries and lime slices for garnish (optional)

Preparation:

• In a blender, combine the fresh raspberries, lime juice, honey or maple syrup, and cold water.

- Blend until smooth.

- Strain the mixture through a fine mesh sieve to remove any pulp (optional).

- Fill glasses halfway with the raspberry-lime mixture.

- Top off your glass with sparkling water.

- Add ice cubes.

- Garnish with fresh raspberries and lime slices if desired.

- Serve immediately and enjoy the bubbly Raspberry Lime Sparkler!

Pineapple Mint Mojito Smoothie:

Ingredients:

- 1 cup chopped pineapple

- Handful of fresh mint leaves

- Juice of 1 lime

- 1 tablespoon honey or maple syrup

- 1/2 cup coconut water

- Ice cubes

- Mint sprigs and the pineapple wedges for garnish (optional)

Preparation:

• In a blender, combine the chopped pineapple, fresh mint leaves, lime juice, honey or maple syrup, and coconut water.

• Blend until smooth.

• Pour the Pineapple Mint Mojito Smoothie into glasses filled with ice cubes.

• Garnish with mint sprigs and pineapple wedges if desired.

• Serve immediately and enjoy the tropical Pineapple Mint Mojito Smoothie!

Strawberry Cucumber Refresher:

Ingredients:

- 1 cup sliced strawberries

- 1/2 cucumber, peeled and chopped

- Handful of fresh mint leaves

- Juice of 1 lime

- 1 tablespoon honey or maple syrup

- 1 cup cold water

- Ice cubes

- Mint sprigs and strawberry slices for garnish (optional)

Preparation:

- In a blender, combine the sliced strawberries, chopped cucumber, fresh mint leaves, lime juice, honey or maple syrup, and cold water.

- Blend until smooth.

- Strain the mixture through a fine mesh sieve to remove any pulp (optional).

- Pour the Strawberry Cucumber Refresher into glasses filled with ice cubes.

- Garnish with mint sprigs and strawberry slices if desired.

- Serve immediately and enjoy the rejuvenating Strawberry Cucumber Refresher!

Green Grape Hydrator:

Ingredients:

- 1 cup green grapes

- Handful of spinach leaves

- Juice of 1 lime

- 1 tablespoon honey or maple syrup

- 1 cup cold water

- Ice cubes

- Lime slices and grape clusters for garnish (optional)

Preparation:

- In a blender, combine the green grapes, spinach leaves, lime juice, honey or maple syrup, and cold water.

- Blend until smooth.

- Strain the mixture through a fine mesh sieve to remove any pulp (optional).

- Pour the Green Grape Hydrator into glasses filled with ice cubes.

- Garnish with lime slices and grape clusters if desired.

- Serve immediately and enjoy the refreshing Green Grape Hydrator!

Peach Basil Quencher:

Ingredients:

- 1 ripe peach, pitted and sliced

- Handful of fresh basil leaves

- Juice of 1 lemon

- 1 tablespoon honey or maple syrup

- 1 cup cold water

- Ice cubes

- Basil leaves and peach slices for garnish (optional)

Preparation:

- In a blender, combine the sliced peach, fresh basil leaves, lemon juice, honey or maple syrup, and cold water.

- Blend until smooth.

- Strain the mixture through a fine mesh sieve to remove any pulp (optional).

- Pour the Peach Basil Quencher into glasses filled with ice cubes.

- Garnish with basil leaves and peach slices if desired.

- Serve immediately and enjoy the delightful Peach Basil Quencher!

Honeydew Melon Mint Chill:

Ingredients:

- 1 cup diced honeydew melon

- Handful of fresh mint leaves

- Juice of 1 lime

- 1 tablespoon honey or maple syrup

- 1 cup cold water

- Ice cubes

- Mint sprigs and honeydew melon balls for garnish (optional)

Preparation:

- In a blender, combine the diced honeydew melon, fresh mint leaves, lime juice, honey or maple syrup, and cold water.

- Blend until smooth.

- Strain the mixture through a fine mesh sieve to remove any pulp (optional).

- Pour the Honeydew Melon Mint Chill into glasses filled with ice cubes.

- Garnish with mint sprigs and honeydew melon balls if desired.

- Serve immediately and enjoy the cooling Honeydew Melon Mint Chill!

Blueberry Lavender Lemonade:

Ingredients:

- 1 cup fresh or frozen blueberries

- 1 tablespoon dried culinary lavender buds

- Juice of 1 lemon

- 1 tablespoon honey or maple syrup

- 1 cup cold water

- Ice cubes

• Fresh blueberries and lavender sprigs for garnish (optional)

Preparation:

• In a blender, combine the blueberries, dried lavender buds, lemon juice, honey or maple syrup, and cold water.

• Blend until smooth.

• Strain the mixture through a fine mesh sieve to remove any pulp (optional).

• Pour the Blueberry Lavender Lemonade into glasses filled with ice cubes.

• Garnish with fresh blueberries and lavender sprigs if desired.

• Serve immediately and enjoy the floral and fruity Blueberry Lavender Lemonade!

Nourishing Afternoon Delights:

Avocado Berry Bliss:

Ingredients:

- 1/2 ripe avocado

- 1/2 cup mixed berries. (strawberries, blueberries, raspberries)

- 1/2 cup spinach leaves

- 1 tablespoon honey or maple syrup

- 1 cup almond milk. (or any milk of your choice)

- Ice cubes

- Fresh berries for garnish (optional)

Preparation:

• Scoop out the flesh of the ripe avocado and place it in a blender.

• Add the mixed berries, spinach leaves, honey or maple syrup, and almond milk to the blender.

• Blend until smooth and creamy.

• If the smoothie is too thick, add more almond milk or ice cubes and blend again until desired consistency is reached.

• Pour the Avocado Berry Bliss into glasses.

• Garnish with fresh berries if desired.

• Serve immediately and enjoy the creamy goodness of this nutritious smoothie!

Spinach Mango Tango:

Ingredients:

- 1 cup chopped mango

- 1/2 cup spinach leaves

- Juice of 1 lime

- 1 tablespoon honey or maple syrup

- 1 cup coconut water

- Ice cubes

- Mango slices for garnish (optional)

Preparation:

- Place the chopped mango, spinach leaves, lime juice, honey or maple syrup, and coconut water in a blender.

- Blend until smooth and well combined.

- If the smoothie is too thick, add more coconut water or ice cubes and blend again until desired consistency is reached.

- Pour the Spinach Mango Tango into glasses.

- Garnish with mango slices if desired.

- Serve immediately and enjoy the tropical flavors of this refreshing smoothie!

Papaya Coconut Dream:

Ingredients:

- 1 cup diced papaya

- 1/2 cup coconut milk

- 1/2 cup coconut water

- 1 tablespoon honey or maple syrup

- 1 teaspoon vanilla extract

- Ice cubes

- Toasted coconut flakes for garnish (optional)

Preparation:

- Place the diced papaya, coconut milk, coconut water, honey or maple syrup, and vanilla extract in a blender.

- Blend until smooth and creamy.

- If the smoothie is too thick, add more coconut water or ice cubes and blend again until desired consistency is reached.

- Pour the Papaya Coconut Dream into glasses.

- Garnish with toasted coconut flakes if desired.

- Serve immediately and enjoy the tropical Papaya Coconut Dream!

Blackberry Almond Joy:

Ingredients:

- 1/2 cup blackberries

- 1/4 cup almonds

- 1/2 ripe banana

- 1 tablespoon cocoa powder

- 1 cup almond milk. (or any milk of your choice)

- Ice cubes

- Blackberries for garnish (optional)

Preparation:

- Place the blackberries, almonds, ripe banana, cocoa powder, and almond milk in a blender.

- Blend until smooth and well combined.

- If the smoothie is too thick, add more almond milk or ice cubes and blend again until desired consistency is reached.

- Pour the Blackberry Almond Joy into glasses.

- Garnish with blackberries if desired.

- Serve immediately and enjoy the rich chocolatey flavor of this delicious smoothie!

Cherry Vanilla Protein Smoothie:

Ingredients:

- 1 cup frozen cherries

- 1/2 cup plain Greek yogurt

- 1 scoop vanilla protein powder

- 1 tablespoon honey or maple syrup

- 1 cup almond milk. (or any milk of your choice)

- Ice cubes

- Fresh cherries for garnish (optional)

Preparation:

● Place the frozen cherries, Greek yogurt, vanilla protein powder, honey or maple syrup, and almond milk in a blender.

● Blend until smooth and creamy.

● If the smoothie is too thick, add more almond milk or ice cubes and blend again until desired consistency is reached.

● Pour the Cherry Vanilla Protein Smoothie into glasses.

● Garnish with fresh cherries if desired.

● Serve immediately and enjoy the protein-packed goodness of this satisfying smoothie!

Fig and Walnut Wonder:

Ingredients:

- 2 ripe figs. Stems removed and quartered

- 1/4 cup walnuts

- 1/2 cup plain Greek yogurt

- 1 tablespoon honey or maple syrup

- 1 cup almond milk. (or any milk of your choice)

- Ice cubes

- Fresh fig slices for garnish (optional)

Preparation:

- Place the ripe figs, walnuts, Greek yogurt, honey or maple syrup, and almond milk in a blender.

- Blend until smooth and well combined.

- If the smoothie is too thick, add more almond milk or ice cubes and blend again until desired consistency is reached.

- Pour the Fig and Walnut Wonder into glasses.

- Garnish with fresh fig slices if desired.

- Serve immediately and enjoy the nutty sweetness of this delightful smoothie!

Green Apple Kiwi Surprise:

Ingredients:

- 1 green apple, cored and chopped

- 2 kiwis, peeled and chopped

- Handful of spinach leaves

- Juice of 1 lime

- 1 tablespoon honey or maple syrup

- 1 cup coconut water

- Ice cubes

- Kiwi slices for garnish (optional)

Preparation:

- Place the chopped green apple, chopped kiwis, spinach leaves, lime juice, honey or maple syrup, and coconut water in a blender.

- Blend until smooth and well combined.

- If the smoothie is too thick, add more coconut water or ice cubes and blend again until desired consistency is reached.

- Pour the Green Apple Kiwi Surprise into glasses.

- Garnish with kiwi slices if desired.

- Serve immediately and enjoy the refreshing tartness of this green smoothie!

Pomegranate Blueberry Delight:

Ingredients:

- 1/2 cup pomegranate seeds

- 1/2 cup blueberries

- 1/2 cup plain Greek yogurt

- 1 tablespoon honey or maple syrup

- 1 cup almond milk. (or any milk of your choice)

- Ice cubes

- Fresh blueberries for garnish (optional)

Preparation:

- Place the pomegranate seeds, blueberries, Greek yogurt, honey or maple syrup, and almond milk in a blender.

- Blend until smooth and creamy.

- If the smoothie is too thick, add more almond milk or ice cubes and blend again until desired consistency is reached.

- Pour the Pomegranate Blueberry Delight into glasses.

- Garnish with fresh blueberries if desired.

- Serve immediately and enjoy the antioxidant-rich goodness of this vibrant smoothie!

Coconut Watermelon Cooler:

Ingredients:

- 1 cup diced watermelon

- 1/2 cup coconut water

- Juice of 1 lime

- 1 tablespoon honey or maple syrup

- Handful of fresh mint leaves

- Ice cubes

- Watermelon wedges for garnish (optional)

Preparation:

- Place the diced watermelon, coconut water, lime juice, honey or maple syrup, and fresh mint leaves in a blender.

- Blend until smooth and well combined.

- If the smoothie is too thick, add more coconut water or ice cubes and blend again until desired consistency is reached.

- Pour the Coconut Watermelon Cooler into glasses.

• Garnish with watermelon wedges if desired.

• Serve immediately and enjoy the hydrating and refreshing Coconut Watermelon Cooler!

Mango Cashew Cream Smoothie:

Ingredients:

• 1 cup diced mango

• 1/4 cup raw cashews

• 1/2 cup plain Greek yogurt

• 1 tablespoon honey or maple syrup

• 1 cup almond milk. (or any milk of your choice)

- Ice cubes

- Cashew pieces for garnish (optional)

Preparation:

- Place the diced mango, raw cashews, Greek yogurt, honey or maple syrup, and almond milk in a blender.

- Blend until smooth and creamy.

- If the smoothie is too thick, add more almond milk or ice cubes and blend again until desired consistency is reached.

- Pour the Mango Cashew Cream Smoothie into glasses.

- Garnish with cashew pieces if desired. Serve immediately and enjoy the rich and creamy Mango Cashew Cream Smoothie!

Soothing Evening Treats: Banana Cinnamon Bedtime Blend:

Ingredients:

- 1 ripe banana

- 1/2 teaspoon ground cinnamon

- 1 tablespoon honey or maple syrup

- 1 cup unsweetened almond milk. (or any milk of your choice)

- Ice cubes (optional)

Preparation:

- Peel the ripe banana and then place it in a blender.

- Add the ground cinnamon, honey or maple syrup, and unsweetened almond milk to the blender.

- Blend until smooth and creamy.

- If desired, add ice cubes to the blender and blend again until well combined.

- Pour the Banana Cinnamon Bedtime Blend into glasses.

- Serve immediately and enjoy this soothing and comforting bedtime treat!

Vanilla Date Nightcap:

Ingredients:

- 2 dates, pitted

- 1 teaspoon vanilla extract

- 1 cup unsweetened almond milk. (or any milk of your choice)

- Ice cubes (optional)

Preparation:

- Place the pitted dates, vanilla extract, and unsweetened almond milk in a blender.

- Blend till the dates are fully incorporated and the mixture is also smooth.

- If desired, add ice cubes to the blender and blend again until well combined.

- Pour the Vanilla Date Nightcap into glasses.

- Serve immediately and enjoy this creamy and naturally sweet nightcap!

Chamomile Peach Relaxer:

Ingredients:

- 1 chamomile tea bag

- 1 ripe peach, pitted and chopped

- 1 tablespoon honey or maple syrup

- 1 cup unsweetened almond milk. (or any milk of your choice)

- Ice cubes (optional)

Preparation:

• Steep the chamomile tea bag in hot water according to package instructions and let it cool completely.

• In a blender, combine the chopped peach, honey or maple syrup, cooled • chamomile tea, and unsweetened almond milk.

• Blend until smooth and well combined.

• If desired, add ice cubes to the blender and blend again until well combined.

• Pour the Chamomile Peach Relaxer into glasses.

• Serve immediately and enjoy this calming and refreshing bedtime beverage!

Lavender Blueberry Dream:

Ingredients:

- 1/2 teaspoon dried culinary lavender buds

- 1/2 cup fresh or frozen blueberries

- 1 tablespoon honey or maple syrup

- 1 cup unsweetened almond milk. (or any milk of your choice)

- Ice cubes (optional)

Preparation:

- In a small saucepan, heat the unsweetened almond milk until warm but not boiling.

- Add the dried culinary lavender buds to the warm almond milk and let it steep for 5-10 minutes.

- Strain the lavender-infused almond milk to remove the lavender buds.

- In a blender, combine the blueberries, honey or maple syrup, and lavender-infused almond milk.

- Blend until smooth and well combined.

- If desired, add ice cubes to the blender and blend again until well combined.

Pour the Lavender Blueberry Dream into glasses.

- Serve immediately and enjoy this fragrant and soothing bedtime treat!

Honeydew Mint Serenity:

Ingredients:

- 1 cup diced honeydew melon

- Handful of fresh mint leaves

- 1 tablespoon honey or maple syrup

- 1 cup unsweetened coconut water

- Ice cubes (optional)

Preparation:

- In a blender, combine the diced honeydew melon, fresh mint leaves, honey or maple syrup, and unsweetened coconut water.

- Blend until smooth and well combined.

- If desired, add ice cubes to the blender and blend again until well combined.

- Pour the Honeydew Mint Serenity into glasses.

- Serve immediately and enjoy this refreshing and hydrating bedtime beverage!

Almond Cherry Slumber Smoothie:

Ingredients:

- 1/2 cup frozen cherries

- 1 tablespoon almond butter

- 1 tablespoon honey or maple syrup

• 1 cup unsweetened almond milk. (or any milk of your choice)

• Ice cubes (optional)

Preparation:

• In a blender, combine the frozen cherries, almond butter, honey or maple syrup, and unsweetened almond milk.

• Blend until smooth and well combined.

If desired, add ice cubes to the blender and blend again until well combined.

• Pour the Almond Cherry Slumber Smoothie into glasses.

• Serve immediately and enjoy this creamy and satisfying bedtime treat!

Passionfruit Sleepytime Soother:

Ingredients:

- Pulp of 1 passionfruit

- 1/2 ripe banana

- 1/2 cup plain Greek yogurt

- 1 tablespoon honey or maple syrup

- 1 cup unsweetened almond milk. (or any milk of your choice)

- Ice cubes (optional)

Preparation:

- Scoop out the pulp of the passionfruit and place it in a blender.

• Add the ripe banana, Greek yogurt, honey or maple syrup, and unsweetened almond milk to the blender.

• Blend until smooth and creamy.

• If desired, add ice cubes to the blender and blend again until well combined.

• Pour the Passionfruit Sleepytime Soother into glasses.

• Serve immediately and enjoy this tropical and soothing bedtime beverage!

Kiwi Coconut Sleep Elixir:

Ingredients:

• 2 kiwis, peeled and chopped

• 1/2 cup coconut milk

- 1 tablespoon honey or maple syrup

- 1/2 teaspoon vanilla extract

- 1 cup unsweetened almond milk. (or any milk of your choice)

- Ice cubes (optional)

Preparation:

- In a blender, combine the chopped kiwis, coconut milk, honey or maple syrup, vanilla extract, and unsweetened almond milk.

- Blend until smooth and well combined.

- If desired, add ice cubes to the blender and blend again until well combined.

- Pour the Kiwi Coconut Sleep Elixir into glasses.

- Serve immediately and enjoy this creamy and tropical bedtime elixir!

Pumpkin Spice Nighttime Nectar:

Ingredients:

- 1/2 cup pumpkin puree

- 1/2 teaspoon pumpkin pie spice

- 1 tablespoon honey or maple syrup

- 1 cup unsweetened almond milk. (or any milk of your choice)

- Ice cubes (optional)

Preparation:

● In a blender, combine the pumpkin puree, pumpkin pie spice, honey or maple syrup, and unsweetened almond milk.

● Blend until smooth and well combined.

If desired, add ice cubes to the blender and blend again until well combined.

● Pour the Pumpkin Spice Nighttime Nectar into glasses.

● Serve immediately and enjoy this cozy and comforting bedtime beverage!

Cardamom Pear Lullaby:

Ingredients:

- 1 ripe pear, peeled and chopped

- 1/4 teaspoon ground cardamom

- 1 tablespoon honey or maple syrup

- 1 cup unsweetened almond milk. (or any milk of your choice)

- Ice cubes (optional)

Preparation:

- In a blender, combine the chopped pear, ground cardamom, honey or maple syrup, and unsweetened almond milk.

- Blend until smooth and well combined.

• If desired, add ice cubes to the blender and blend again until well combined.

• Pour the Cardamom Pear Lullaby into glasses.

• Serve immediately and enjoy this fragrant and soothing bedtime blend!

Conclusion

"Diabetic Renal Smoothie Cookbook for Beginners" offers a comprehensive guide to creating delicious and nutritious smoothies tailored specifically for individuals managing both diabetes and renal health concerns. Throughout this cookbook, we've explored a wide range of smoothie recipes that prioritize ingredients that support blood sugar management and kidney function, while also delivering on taste and convenience.

Smoothies are a convenient way to incorporate nutrient-rich ingredients into your diet, providing essential vitamins, minerals, and antioxidants that support overall health and well-being. By focusing on ingredients with low glycemic indexes and kidney-friendly properties, these smoothie recipes offer a flavorful way to manage blood sugar levels and support renal function.

Whether you're looking for a quick and easy breakfast option, a satisfying snack, or a refreshing beverage to enjoy any time of day, the recipes in this cookbook provide a variety of options so to suit your taste preferences and your dietary needs. From fruity blends to creamy concoctions, there's something for everyone to enjoy.

By incorporating these smoothies into your daily routine, you can take proactive steps towards better managing your diabetes and supporting your kidney health. With a focus on balance, variety, and moderation, these recipes offer a delicious way to nourish your body and promote overall wellness.

We hope this cookbook inspires you to get creative in the kitchen and discover the joy of crafting delicious and healthful smoothies that support your unique health journey. Cheers to good health and happy blending!